Book 1

Coconut Oil for Easy Weight Loss

BY LINDSEY P

&

Book 2

The Beginners Guide to Medicinal Plants

BY LINDSEY P

Book 1

Coconut Oil for Easy Weight Loss

BY LINDSEY P

A Step by Step Guide for Using Virgin Coconut Oil for Quick and Easy Weight Loss

3RD Edition

Essential Oils Box Set #30: Coconut Oil for Easy Weight Loss & The Beginners
Guide to Medical Plants

Table Of Contents

Introduction

I want to thank you and congratulate you for purchasing the ebook, *"Coconut Oil For Easy Weight Loss: A Step-By-Step Guide For Using Virgin Coconut Oil For Quick And Easy Weight Loss"*.

This book contains information on how Virgin Coconut Oil benefits our bodies as well as the different means through which it can hasten our weight loss. It is quite unconventional, considering that oil typically equals fat when we think about it. However, this is certainly not the case with coconut oil for it contains many beneficial nutrients that are good for our bodies—inside and out.

Here, you'll be provided with more than just simple facts. You'll also be given a few recipes that you can enjoy during your diet without having to worry that you'll end up ruining your routine. In fact, by eating these, you'll lose weight more efficiently.

Thanks again for purchasing this book. I hope you enjoy it!

Chapter 1: What is Virgin Coconut Oil?

Conventional thought used to consider different fats such as coconut oil to be just as unhealthy as animal fat and that consuming it would eventually lead to heart disease. However, we have since discovered that this is not true at all, and that coconut oil is actually very healthy for our cardiac system. It is quite unique. So what sets it apart from other oils? From food products such as butter and lard, which are also used for cooking but carries with it major health risks.

So what's in a coconut?

Coconuts, despite their humble appearance are actually excellent sources of nutrition. It can also be considered as a complete food with its healthy meat, oil and juice. Did you know that there are people who survive on nothing but the coconut? That's how great this often overlooked fruit is. Arguably, it's the oil that is the most nutritious and beneficial part of the fruit. With over 90% saturated fat (the good kind) content along with antifungal, antimicrobial and antibacterial properties, it's no wonder people use it from cooking to healing.

How does Virgin Coconut Oil differ from other types of coconut oils?

What you must first know is that most commercial grade coconut oils are actually derived from copra or dried coconut meat. This can be made through various means such as sun drying, kiln drying as well as smoke drying. If dried coconut meat is used for the base material, the unrefined oil from it would not be fit for human consumption, at least not after it has been purified—or refined. This is because dried coconut meat can be very unsanitary considering the process through which it is made. The standard product derived from copra is called RBD coconut oil. RBD stands for refined, bleached and deodorized. There are chemicals used to make it.

On the other hand, virgin coconut oil or VCO, is derived from fresh coconut meat; hence, it retains the scent and taste of the actual coconut. In fact, this is one of the ways through which you'd be able to differentiate it from an RBD. Because of the fact that it hasn't been processed and was derived through a sanitary manner, virgin coconut oil is considered to be much healthier and safer when it comes to human consumption. It must also be noted that it also retains far more of the good, healthy stuff that has made coconut oil a popular functional food by the medical community as well as health-conscious people all over the world.

More recently, however, it's being recognized for its effectiveness when it comes to hastening weight loss in people as well as lowering risks of heart disease development.

Medium Chain Fatty Acids (MCFA's)

A great majority of the fats that we consume are actually long chain fatty acids that the body needs to break down before we're able to absorb the nutrients we need from it. This takes a lot of work. On the other hand, the coconut oil contains high amounts of short and medium chain fatty acids which can be directly digested and sent to the liver in order to produce more energy for the body's use.

If you have diabetes, this is good for you as well. Because the MCFAs are sent directly to the liver, there is no need for our bodies to produce pancreatic enzymes or bile in order to digest it. This is one of the reasons why many experts recommend it for diabetics.

As for easy and efficient weight loss, the MCFA's serve a purpose as well.

MCFA's can, in fact, boost our metabolism along with our energy. So if you're exercising, this would provide you with a great advantage as you won't get tired easily. You'll also be able to quickly burn the food you eat and turn that into energy as well, enough to get you through the day or the exercise routines you intend to do.

What About Saturated Fat? Isn't that unhealthy?

Still concerned about this? While it does have quite the bad rep, it is worth considering that not all saturated fats are actually bad for the body. This is because they don't behave in the same way once we've consumed it. Take coconut oil for example. Because of its high Lauric acid content, it actually does more good than bad for us. This is apparent in the diets of many Thai people. They consume large amounts of saturated fats such as coconut oil and yet, they also have the lowest average when it comes to heart risk when compared to other countries.

Chapter 2: How Virgin Coconut Oil Works For Weight Loss

There are many negative connotations when it comes to coconut oil and it's very generous saturated fat content, but fortunately all of those old beliefs have been debunked. These days, people no longer avoid consuming and using coconut oil because they are more aware of its health benefits and among those—weight loss.

The trick is simple: Coconut oil helps in boosting our metabolism thus allowing our bodies to burn fat quicker and more efficiently.

Some people who want to lose weight use thermogenic stimulants. These are basically drugs that produce heat through metabolic stimulation. A higher metabolic rate means that the body burns fat faster. People who have high metabolic rates usually don't have to worry about eating too much food because their body easily burns off the fats and leave very little to be stored in the body. Consequently, they also tend to have a slimmer figure because their bodies do not store excess fat.

However, with all the known dangers that are typically associated with thermogenic stimulants, it's not surprising that a lot of people tend to simply stay away from them. For people who are watching their weight, this is an unfortunate thing because it does help them improve their metabolic rate. Luckily, they now have another alternative. Something more natural that wouldn't have them resorting to weight loss pills or overdosing on caffeine just to get the same effect. Extra virgin coconut oil is one of the safest options when it comes to losing weight quickly.

Effect on metabolism

Earlier, we learned that coconut oil primarily consists of short and medium-chain fatty acids and these are known to help in speeding up our metabolic rate. Metabolism is the body's energy expenditure. Energy expenditure is the rate at which calories are consumed. If a person has a high metabolic rate, then the rate of energy consumption is also increased. Thus, adding virgin coconut oil to any food will lessen the effective number of calories found in the meal. In fact, according to a study, energy expenditure in an average weighted individual can be increased by up to 48%, meaning metabolism increased by 48%. If a person is obese, the energy expenditure can be up to 60%. The heavier a person is, the greater the effect of virgin coconut oil to increase the rate of metabolism. The study also showed that contrary to what some people believe, the effects lasted for 24 hours maximum. Virgin coconut oil is easily digestible and could be turned to energy without much trouble. This is a significant find, considering, the biggest disadvantage that many weight watchers have is a slow metabolism brought on by years of eating unhealthy food. If they are able to change that, well, the process itself should be much easier and quicker to accomplish.

There are other ways through which coconut oil can help when it comes to weight loss and maintaining a healthy weight. Below are a few examples:

1. Coconut oil helps in slowing down the digestion of our food and this can help us feel much fuller after a meal. If you add coconut oil to your diet, you can also help reduce the need to snack in between meals because you won't feel hungry easily. This helps you avoid overeating as well.

2. Because of its ability to help slow down the process of digestion, coconut oil can also help in preventing blood sugar fluctuations that tend to happen after we've eaten a rather heavy meal. So if you have a tendency to feel sleepy after lunch, consuming coconut oil together with your meal would allow you to avoid that.

3. The medium chain fatty acids found in coconut oil is also capable of destroying Candida which is a condition wherein there's yeast overgrowth in the body. This would actually trigger weight gain as well as a craving for carbohydrates as well as induce fatigue. If you want to lose weight successfully, you need to eliminate this first. Only then will you be able to maintain your desired weight.

4. For detoxifying the body, coconut oil is also a great product to use. It helps in ridding the body of many infirmities as well as in balancing our digestive tract all while nourishing the healthy cells in our bodies. This simple process can help in restoring our body to its previous health while paving the way for a quick and easy weight loss.

5. Virgin coconut oil helps curb the cravings for sweets. Eating sweets is one of the hardest things to give up. For most people, it is the ultimate test of their will power. Many diets fail because people fail to curb their craving for sugary foods. But here's a solution. When you feel the urge to eat something sweet, take a teaspoon of virgin coconut oil instead. Consume it with a slice of meat, yogurt, cheese, or any food, and the craving should go away.

Produces Energy and Not Fat

Whenever people go on diets as a means of losing weight, they would typically restrain themselves from eating foods which are known to contain the most amount of fat. But why is it singled out? Other than the fact that it increases the calories in our body, it is because of the way it is digested and used that contributes to the most amount of fat storage. Simply put, the fat we eat is also the fat that ends up on the thicker parts of our bodies.

Whenever we eat fat, it is broken down by the body into individual fatty acids and then bundled up into fat and protein called lipoproteins. These are then sent into our bloodstream where the fatty acids are directly deposited into our fat cells.

Other nutrients such as protein and carbohydrate are also broken down but unlike the fatty acids, they are immediately utilized for energy or the building of body tissue. Only when we eat in excess of those two does it become converted into body fat.

MCFA's found in virgin coconut oil are digested and utilized differently, however. Unlike typical food fat, they are not bundled into lipoproteins or circulated in the bloodstream before ending up in storage (in your arms, thighs and tummy). Rather, they are actually converted into energy immediately much like the protein and carbs that you consume. So when you consume virgin coconut oil, you gain more energy without having to worry about the fat getting stored in your body. This has been a well-documented fat that's been observed in both animals and humans. The research clearly shows that by replacing your usual oil with the virgin coconut variety, you will be able to decrease your body weight as well as reduce the amount of stored fat in your body.

Low-fat diets versus fat in VCO

How about low-fat diets which are so popular these days? Why is the virgin coconut oil weight loss more effective than simply reducing fat intake? This is because low-fat diets do not provide a long-term solution to weight loss. It does not help you lose weight permanently. It will only allow you to lose weight for the duration that you are on the diet, and most of the time, this means starving yourself. Most low-fat diet makes people cranky, moody and miserable because they are always hungry. They limit what they eat, something that any person cannot do for an extended period of time. There will be a breaking point, and when they do start to eat normally again, they gain back all the pounds.

The thing is, people need fat in their diets in order to get the feeling of satisfaction. In fact, people who eat fat generally eat less. The less a person eats the lesser calories they consume. But we're not talking about the usual fat people get from cooking oil, meat and butter. We're talking about the good kind of fat that is not dangerous to consume, such as the fat in virgin coconut oil. It has gained a reputation for being the world's only natural low-calorie fat. This means that you can eat the same types of food but when virgin coconut oil is added to the meal, less calories are consumed.

Earlier we have learned that the fat contained in virgin coconut oil is not the bad stuff. It is the healthy kind of fat which is easily digested by the body and converts into energy, instead of being stored in the body. The body needs an adequate amount of fat in order for weight loss to become permanent. The fat in virgin coconut oil helps people feel satisfied and full after a meal, thus, they have lesser hunger pangs and reduces appetite on the next meal. They have a lesser tendency to eat snacks and eat less during meals. The result is lower overall fat consumption. This is because the fat helps to slow down the emptying of the stomach, which allows a person to feel full much longer. Lesser meals mean lesser calories consumed during the day, and consequently, less fat stored in the body.

This fact is actually backed up by studies, one of which is published in the Journal of Nutrition. In the study, researchers demonstrated that diets containing medium-chain triglycerides (MCTs) such as those found in coconut oil can help increase energy, speed up metabolism, decrease appetite, burn calories faster, lower fat mass in the body and decrease overall weight. Thus, virgin coconut oil has been recommended for the treatment of obesity.

How VCO will help if you are obese

Obesity is the number one problem being faced by many individuals today. The incidence of obesity is even more significant in the Western part of the world wherein access to coconut products is limited compared to tropical countries wherein coconuts grow prolifically. How will you know if you are already considered obese? There's a difference between being overweight and being obese. Being overweight means you have a Body Mass Index (BMI) of between 25 to 29. Having a BMI of 30 and higher means you are already considered obese. This means that your weight has already reached a dangerous level that it is already being detrimental to your health. Obesity is linked to cardiovascular diseases, diabetes and joint problems, among other diseases.

For obese people the recommendation is usually to limit fat consumption. One gram of fat can supply double the amount of protein as well as carbohydrate-rich foods, for the same number of calories. This means the need to go on a diet. However, hunger is usually the number one problem faced by obese people while on a diet. The solution is to eat more foods that has lower calories and can easily fill you up to satisfy the hunger.

This is where the virgin coconut oil comes in. This is a low-calorie fat that can help people with weight problems lose their excess pounds. It has less calories than other fats, however, it still has a higher calorie content compared to protein and carbohydrates. This means that it has the ability to satisfy hunger compared to carbohydrates and protein. When food is taken with virgin coconut oil, it takes longer for the body to feel hungry until the next meal. Thus, the person will eat fewer meals within the day. There will be fewer urges to munch on snacks. Add this to the stimulating effect virgin coconut oil has on the metabolism. It increases the rate of burn of calories in the body. As long as you don't overeat, the virgin coconut oil can stimulate metabolism more effectively.

Will VCO make skinny people even thinner?

Just because virgin coconut oil has the ability to reduce the amount of fat in the body, it doesn't mean that it will make skinny people even skinnier. According to studies, if a person has little body fat, the coconut oil will have a lesser effect in firing up the metabolism and burning calories. In fact, people who are underweight or are considered malnourished can actually gain some weight. Virgin coconut oil will help the body reach its ideal weight that is optimal for the healthy functioning of the entire body. Thus, skinny people can still reap the health benefits of virgin coconut oil and should not be afraid to continue taking it.

Chapter 3: Starting Your VCO Weight Loss Regimen

Using virgin coconut oil diet to lose weight is not just about taking a few doses of oil daily. It is not a drug that will magically help you lose weight while maintaining poor eating habits and a sedentary lifestyle. The decision to lose weight using coconut oil is all about revolutionizing one's health and switching to a healthier way of eating and living. So be prepared to embrace a few good things and get rid of all the unhealthy negative stuff. Let's start with the food.

Food

If intending to lose weight with virgin coconut oil, here are some of the foods to avoid:

1. Processed vegetable oils

2. Hydrogenated vegetable oils such as margarine and shortening

3. Overly processed grains such as white bread, white rice, cereals, crackers, etc.

4. Pasteurized and homogenized milk

5. Sugar and sweets

Basically, stay away from all junk foods, anything artificial and all kinds of processed foods. It is best to eat more fruits and vegetables daily. Just how much fruits and vegetables should one eat? Typically, it is recommended to get at least 5 servings of fruits throughout the day and even more vegetables. However, recent studies are showing that 9 servings a day will be most beneficial to health.

No need to diet. Rejoice in the fact that there's no need to go on a diet and munch on carrot sticks all the time. It is not necessary to reduce the amount of food eaten either. What needs to be done is to replace the kind of food being eaten and add coconut oil to it. Go ahead and enjoy your chicken, but remove the skin which contains the most fat and cook the white meat in coconut oil. Craving for ice cream? Go ahead! But try the yummy yogurt sorbet instead and mix in coconut oil to it. Stir fry vegetables in virgin coconut oil and top it on fried rice.

If you are accustomed to snacking on a burger meal or a bag of chips, try replacing it with a variety of fruits you love to eat. The cost will probably be the same, or even cheaper if the fruits are in season. Eat a lot more raw and cooked vegetables. Examples of vegetables that can be eaten raw include cucumber, lettuce and carrots.

Learn to cook. Another thing that would be helpful is for you to learn how to cook. Eating out can be a real fancy treat. There's no harm in dining out every once in a while. However, food cooked commercially usually contains transfat and gluten. Majority of what you eat should still be home cooked in order to incorporate virgin coconut oil into the dish.

Keep a list of quick and easy VCO recipes. Yes, we know, cooking can be quite a chore, especially if you have to wash the dirty dished and the sink afterwards. But there are ways to make cooking easier by planning meals. Start by collecting various recipes that includes virgin coconut oil. Compile it in a notebook or save in the computer for a quick reference. Plan your meals so that you will cook and prepare only once and it would be good enough for the whole day, or even a few days. There's no need to cook several times a day. Some cooked meals can be placed in the refrigerator and reheated when needed. Keep healthy snacks in the fridge such as cut up fruits and yogurt. Stock the pantry with healthy snacks such as wheat bread, organic sugarless peanut butter, nuts and seeds. And of course, always stock up on bottles of virgin coconut oil. Keep in within reach all the time.

Exercise

There's no specific exercise necessary to lose weight with virgin coconut oil. What's important is to maintain an active lifestyle. Go to the gym, ride a bike, go swimming, take up sport - basically do anything that will keep you off the couch and on your toes several minutes a day. Choose physical activities that you love to do so that it won't feel like a chore. Not only will it help speed up metabolism, it will also fight off stress. Studies show that even 15 to 30 minutes of brisk walking everyday will significantly help improve health and keep the cardiovascular system circulating properly.

The trick here is to maintain a regular exercise regimen. This means that if you plan to go to the gym at least three days a week, stay on schedule and don't keep changing your routine. If you are not used to exercising regularly, give the body enough time to adjust to the routine. Maintaining regular exercise schedule will allow the muscles to get used to the strain, thus improving the body's strength and endurance to become even more physically active.

One great advantage of taking virgin coconut oil is that it doesn't only help the body lose weight, it also significantly increases energy. That's why maintaining a regular physical activity will be much easier because the body won't feel sluggish.

Avoiding vices

Yes, we're talking about smoking and drinking. If you want to lose weight you should quit it right now and here's why.

Your favorite alcoholic beverage probably contains lots of calories. Studies have shown that there is a 20% increase in calories when an alcoholic beverage is consumed before a meal. A 12 oz beer for example, will contain about 100-150 calories. And let's face it; you don't usually drink just one bottle of beer. A typical drinker would have 2 or more bottles. Your favorite cocktail will contain even more. 4 ounces of Frozen Daiquiri would be about 216 calories, a 4-ounce Margarita is around 270 calories, while a 4 ounces Mai Tai would contain a whopping 310 calories. Add in the side orders of chips other beer-match food and there goes your belly fat.

Smoking on the other hand, is said to actually increase metabolic rate. When a smoker inhales, it makes the heart beat about 10 to 20 times faster per minute, thus increasing a person's metabolic rate. You would probably think, hey this is a good thing for weight loss, right? Not necessarily, because it is at the expense of you developing heart disease, cancer and other smoking-related illnesses. Smoking causes too much stress on the heart. When a smoker suddenly quits, they tend to gain weight because the heart rate slows down, which consequently slows down the rate of metabolism. That is why most people gain weight after quitting smoking. That being said, virgin coconut oil is the perfect solution to help get the metabolic rate back up and running.

Rate of weight loss

The rate in which you will lose weight largely depends on your overall health status, diet and lifestyle. Some people have reported losing more than 50 pounds in a year by simply adding virgin coconut oil to their diet. Others complain that they are not losing enough weight with virgin coconut oil. If you still continue to eat donuts, pizza, burgers and sweets, then the virgin coconut oil is not at fault. It also depends on the person's level of activity. If you are eating healthy, yet continue to live a sedentary lifestyle, then the rate of weight loss will be extremely slow. In order to achieve the optimal result in weight loss, virgin coconut oil should be taken with a sensible diet and a regular physical activity.

Weight loss through virgin coconut oil also depends on your rate of metabolism. Some people lose weight faster because their fast metabolism is inherited. It is in their genes. Men, for example, burn more calories compared to women, even at rest. Age can also be a factor. If you are over 40 years old, your metabolism tends to slow down significantly. To aid virgin coconut oil in firing up your metabolism, keep hydrated by increasing your intake of water and other healthy juices.

What to expect

Remember that using virgin coconut oil will do two major things to help you lose weight – suppress hunger and increase metabolism. The oil will help the body shed body fat at a steady pace each week. Don't expect an overnight result. If coupled with a healthy diet and a good exercise plan, weight loss should be visible within a few months.

Essential Oils Box Set #30: Coconut Oil for Easy Weight Loss & The Beginners Guide to Medical Plants

The physical effect of virgin coconut oil will be very different for each person. Some people have reported losing a lot of the belly fat, which is the hardest kind of fat to burn in the body. Some testimonies say that their weight loss was not visibly significant, but there have been some redistribution of weight in the body and they can suddenly fit into their old pair of jeans. With continued use, virgin coconut oil should be able to help you reach your ideal weight without much effort.

Expect some side effects. This will include loose stools, headaches, nausea, vomiting and possible some rashes. These side effects might happen because the digestive system will adjust to the virgin coconut oil. Remember that aside from weight loss, virgin coconut oil also has a cleansing effect. It is a natural laxative that gets rid of all the toxins in the body. Some people might experience these side effects while others won't. It all depends on how toxic the body is. The virgin coconut oil will initially expel all the toxins in the body before it works its magic. Find out more about virgin coconut oil precautions in the following chapters.

Aside from weight loss, also expect some good changes in energy levels. You will notice this through your daily activities. Some people find themselves still full of energy when arriving home even after an exhausting day at work. Some are happy to have so much extra energy that they are able to perform better and train longer in sports and other physical activities. Higher energy levels also mean lesser fatigue and being mentally alert.

On the physical aspect, virgin coconut oil has amazing effect on the skin and hair. People using virgin coconut oil regularly seem to have healthier looking hair and skin. Their skin seems to look soft and moisturized all the time. Try applying virgin coconut oil topically too to reap its full benefits. Know more about the benefits of using virgin coconut oil on hair and skin in the following chapters.

Chapter 4: Your Daily Dose of VCO

When planning to lose weight using coconut oil, the most common question asked by most people is how much VCO should they take daily? The answer is very vague because there's actually no specific dosage. The real trick is to try to incorporate coconut oil in almost everything you eat, as much as the body can take comfortably. Even taking only half a teaspoon of VCO daily can still have benefits to the body.

Recommended dosage

Generally, the recommended dosage for an average sized adult is to take at least 3 ½ tablespoons a day. Average adult size means a person who weighs around 150 pounds. How did they come to this recommended dosage? This dosage contains the amount of medium-chain fatty acids found in human breast milk. 3 ½ tablespoons contains the amount of MCFA an infant received from the mother's breast milk. This amount of MCFA is what provides complete nutrition and protects the infant from infectious illness. Thus, 3 to 4 tablespoons a day is enough for an adult who weighs 150 pounds. If the weight is less than 150, take ½ tablespoons less for every 25 pounds less the weight. For those who weigh more than 150 pounds, 4 tablespoons is usually enough for the entire day. This dosage however, is not taken all at once. It is best to spread this amount throughout the day.

No strict rules

This dosage however is just a general guideline. There's no need to strictly follow this rule or dosage. A person can take 1 tablespoon a day and it should be enough. There are other means to reap the benefits of coconut oil such as rubbing it all over the body as a moisturizing lotion or using it on the hair to moisturize strands. The important thing is to take the amount most comfortable to consume. Some people are not able to ingest large amounts of fat (even coconut oil) in the body. They tend to have side effects such as nausea and stomach problems caused by loose stools. However, there is no danger posed in consuming too much coconut oil. It basically considered a food, not a drug, so any amount would be safe to consume.

To be safe, start from a small dosage, even just 1 teaspoon a day. Increase the dosage every few days to allow the body to adjust and become accustomed to the oil. Allow the oil to balance the intestinal environment before increasing the dosage. One sign that the digestive tract is still not balanced is when loose stools are experienced. When this happens, stay at a low dose. Your body will tell you if it is ready to increase dosage. Weight loss can be achieved at dosage as long as the oil is incorporated in the diet properly.

Adding coconut oil to the diet

The best way to enjoy virgin coconut oil, especially for those who are not a fan of how it tastes, is to add it to food. Here are some great ways to consume it without gagging every time you take it by the spoonful.

Mix virgin coconut oil with warm drinks. Virgin coconut oil can be added to warm drinks such as hot cocoa, coffee and tea. Warm drinks can help the oil liquefy as virgin coconut oil has a tendency to be solid in consistency, especially during cold weather or when stored in a cool area.

Pour it on top of salads. Instead of the typical olive oil, try using virgin coconut oil on your salads. This will give the salad a little nutty taste.

Use it on stir fry dishes. Stir fried dishes with organic brown rice is one of the best meals to eat when trying to lose weight. It would be even better when the oil used is virgin coconut oil to stir fry the ingredients. Stir frying using virgin coconut oil will give the dish a distinct Asian taste which is delicious!

For frying and sautéing. If you're currently using commercial grade cooking oil to fry your food, get rid of it and replace it with virgin coconut oil instead. You can sauté vegetables, as well as fry meat and fish using virgin coconut oil. Deep frying however, is a different story because virgin coconut oil can be costly to be used often for deep frying. Another alternative would be to use olive oil for that purpose which is also considered healthy oil.

Mix it with sauces and dips. If you're a fan of sauces and dips such as salsa and soy sauce, try adding a tablespoon of virgin coconut oil to it. It will spice up the flavor of your sauces and at the same time, you will be consuming the oil without even noticing it.

Pour it on any food. There's no need to whip up a dish every time just to incorporate virgin coconut oil into your food. Simply pour it over what you're currently eating. Pour a tablespoon over your taco, burrito, sandwich, rice topping - practically any food. Just make sure what you're eating is healthy. You can't pour it over a burger meal and expect the burger to magically become calorie-free.

Mix it with cold food or drinks. Even though the consistency of virgin coconut oil will be in a hard, solid state during the cold season, it can still be added to cold food or drinks. Simply warm the oil first before mixing it with cold foods such as yogurt, ice cream or cold desserts. Just make sure that the dessert is healthy and low in sugar such as fruit salads (without cream).

Here are different ways on how to warm the virgin coconut oil.

1. Place hot water on a cup and let it sit for a minute or two. Then remove the water from the cup and pour in the solid virgin coconut oil. Let it melt in the warm cup while swirling the oil so that it will melt faster, allowing the oil to melt in the warmth of the cup.

2. Place the solid virgin coconut oil on a tablespoon. Place the spoon over the steam of boiling water until it melts.

3. A bottle of virgin coconut oil placed in room temperature will usually stay in liquid state. Unless of course it is winter time and its freezing cold outside. Place the bottle or jar of virgin coconut oil in warm (not hot!) water for a few minutes and allow it to liquefy.

Storing the coconut oil in the refrigerator is not necessary because it has a very long shelf life, even when stored in room temperature only. A room temperature of 77 up to 79 degrees Fahrenheit and lower, the virgin coconut oil will be in a solid state. Temperature 79 degrees Fahrenheit and higher will keep the oil in its liquid state. The oil will look clear as water when in liquid state and a pasty white color when in solid state. The clarity of the oil however, will largely depend on the process in which the virgin coconut oil was produced.

How to buy a high quality virgin coconut oil

When buying coconut oil in the market, you might be faced with different bottles having different brands and labeled with things such as 'refined', 'extra virgin', 'hydrogenated', 'expeller-pressed', 'cold-pressed', etc. Of course you will want the best and comes in the most natural form. So which one is the best for weight loss?

Much of this has already been discussed in the first chapter. There will be two broad categories of coconut oil in the market – refined coconut oil and virgin coconut oil. Refined or RBD (refined, bleached, deodorized) are the ones that are mass produced in an industrial level and is made from copra. Virgin coconut oil is derived from fresh coconuts and this is the one you should look for. This is an oil that has been subjected to less refining. When buying coconut oil, choose the one that has the words 'virgin', 'organic', 'raw' or 'extra virgin' printed in the label.

The thing about these labels is that there is still no worldwide certifying body for coconut oils that would certify that a product is indeed classified as 'virgin'. This means that any manufacturer can use the term 'virgin' or 'extra virgin' and place it on the labels of their products. That is why it is important to choose local brands that have a good reputation and is being sold by reputable supermarkets, health shops and drugstores. Investigate whether the coconut oil is indeed derived from fresh coconuts and not copra, because this is the only way to get the full benefits of virgin coconut oil. Another way to check if the oil is indeed natural and not RBD is if it has a distinct nutty coconut smell. Most people will love the taste and smell of coconut oil. Those who say they don't like how it smells and taste may have used a cheap or poor quality brand.

Chapter 5: Precautions with VCO Use

For a long time, coconut oil has been criticized for being labeled as a saturated fat. People were afraid to use it because it was thought to cause heart problems and can clog the arteries. People assumed that all saturated fats were harmful. It is only now that coconut oil is slowly being accepted again, after recent studies have shown that it is actually not harmful, but on the contrary, highly beneficial and can even fight off heart disease. Still, there are some people who question its benefits, even if evidence has already been shown. More than anything, some are scared of the side effects it brings, especially for those consuming it for the first time. But are these side effects really harmful?

Just because virgin coconut oil is generally healthy, it doesn't mean that it will not come with adverse effects to some people. The effects of coconut oil for weight loss and how fast its benefits will show greatly depend on the person's overall health and how their body will react to it. Some people have low tolerance when ingesting oils that's why they tend to vomit. Others develop rashes because they are simply allergic to it. However, not all reactions to virgin coconut oil means it is a bad effect. More often than not, it signifies how toxic the body is. Virgin coconut oil has detoxifying properties that improves overall health.

Here are some common problems people encounter when taking virgin coconut oil and some ways to resolve it.

Allergic reaction

Coconut can be a source of problem such as allergies. Some people can be allergic to different types of food, animals, and would you believe, even water! There are a lot of weird allergies that actually exist such as allergic reaction to sunlight, cellphones, heat, cold, lettuce, apples, and even their own sweat. Some people might simply be allergic to coconuts in general, and that may include coconut oil. There are some reports of people breaking out into a rash when ingesting coconut oil or even applying it to their skin topically. This allergic reaction may be one of two things. The first one is that the coconut oil is actually working to expel the toxins in the body. In most cleansing and detoxifying process, things can get worst initially before it gets better. If this is the case, the rashes should clear out on its own in a day or two without getting any worse. If the rashes persist, it might be a confirmed allergic reaction to coconuts.

If you have certain allergies to food, it is recommended to first take a test if you are allergic to coconuts. To test, dab a small amount of coconut oil or coconut milk on the forearm. Rub it gently into the skin until it is completely absorbed. Do not wash the area for at least a day and wait to see if your body will have a reaction. The typical sign that you are allergic to coconuts is if the area becomes red or swollen or if you break out into rashes. The body will react with only one application so there's no need to repeat the process. If there is no significant reaction, then you are not allergic to coconuts.

People who are allergic to most nuts do not mean that they are automatically allergic to coconuts. A coconut is basically not categorized as a nut but as a fruit. This fruit is considered to be a very low allergy risk food. People who are allergic to coconut is rare. Coconuts are relatively considered safe to consume except for babies less than a year old. Giving babies coconut oil too early should be done with caution. Watch out for possible allergies and the loose bowel effects. Virgin coconut oil however, does wonderful things to a baby's skin when applied topically. It can heal common skin conditions such as rashes, dry skin, relieve itchiness and soothe insect bites.

If the coconut allergy test reveals you are positive for allergy, then the coconut oil diet is not recommended as it may cause more harm than good. Further consultation with a doctor should be sought.

Loose bowels

The most common reaction people experience when consuming virgin coconut oil is having loose bowels. This usually happens when too much virgin coconut oil is ingested that the body is not accustomed to. The symptoms can be similar to someone experiencing diarrhea or mild food poisoning. Some people report experiencing nausea, vomiting, weakness and frequent bowel movements. For those experiencing constipation, this can be a good thing. But for those who find the symptoms too disturbing, here's what they can do. Instead of consuming the virgin coconut oil purely by the spoonful, try to mix it with food to lessen the ill effect. Decrease the dosage being taken. For example, instead of taking 3 to 4 tablespoons a day, make it 1 to 2 tablespoons. Increase the dosage only when the body has already adjusted to the oil and the digestive system has already normalized and stopped reacting to it. This reaction may just be part of the 'healing crisis' some people undergo while the virgin coconut oil restores their body back to health. Read on to know more about the 'healing crisis' or the healing period.

Healing period

Be aware that aside from helping you lose weight, virgin coconut oil has a restorative effect on the health. That is why some symptoms such as having loose bowels can be experienced. This is not necessarily a negative effect. Many people wonder why they start to feel awful after starting to take virgin coconut oil, when it is supposed to make them feel more energized and revitalized. This can be part of what is called the period of healing crisis. They call it 'healing crisis' because a person's condition may get worse before it gets better. For example, when using virgin coconut oil to treat acne, the acne usually becomes worse first before the skin eventually clears up. This is because the oil is expelling all the toxins in the skin from the pore. It is killing all the bacteria that are causing the breakouts in the first place. When all the bacteria have died out, the skin will become smoother and clearer.

Essential Oils Box Set #30: Coconut Oil for Easy Weight Loss & The Beginners Guide to Medical Plants

People who are trying to lose weight using virgin coconut oil might experience some health setbacks for a few days, especially if their body is overly toxic. Some people will react even to a single teaspoon of virgin coconut oil. This should be taken positively. It is not the oil that is at fault, it is the troubled digestive system. The virgin coconut oil will work to clean up and clear up the toxins from the body, particularly the digestive tract. This cleansing is necessary in order for the weight loss to take place.

Is this normal? Yes it is. The body needs to expel the toxins, it won't die naturally from within you. These are toxins which may have been buried in the body for years. If you study the excretory system, some of the ways in which the body will expel toxins is through bowels and through the skin. These are poisons that are pulled out from the tissues and carried into the bloodstream, then removed by the body's channels of elimination. This is the reason why certain discomforts can manifest. As the body gets rid of the toxins and becomes stronger, it will reach a level wherein it can already tolerate the coconut oil and the symptoms will eventually go away.

Depending on the person's condition, some symptoms that might be experienced are nausea, fatigue, feeling sluggish, diarrhea-like symptoms, vomiting, muscle aches and pains, headache, rashes, fever, mood swings, depression, loss of appetite and many other possible symptoms. When something feels wrong and different after starting to take the virgin coconut oil, it might be associated to the healing effects of coconut oil. Observe these symptoms for a few days because it should eventually go away. When rashes break out however, see if it is an allergic reaction to coconut as previously discussed.

Can I take medication to ease symptoms during the healing period?

Taking medication to ease the symptoms is usually not recommended as it might obstruct the healing effect of the virgin coconut oil. Unless the symptoms are extremely intolerable, it is recommended to use natural pacifying methods such as getting a lot of rest, drinking lots of water, or herbal teas. Symptoms should only last for a day or two. Some people who have more toxins in their bodies can experience the symptoms for several days up to a week. Do not be afraid as this will do your body more good than harm. Get plenty of rest and allow the oil to take its healing effect on you. The symptoms will lessen eventually and the body will feel rejuvenated and more energized than before. However, if symptoms persist for more than this period, and even after reducing the dosage, discontinue use and consult a doctor. A bigger health problem might be causing the side effects.

Chapter 6: Other Known Health Benefits

Besides aiding in speedy weight loss, virgin coconut oil has a number of other health benefits. Among them are the following:

1. Alzheimer's and Other Neurological Diseases – The MCT's or medium chain triglycerides commonly found in virgin coconut oil are known to be helpful when it comes to improving our brain function.

2. Anti-aging – It is more effective than chemical-laden creams and lotions when it comes to smoothing out wrinkles, restoring the elasticity of saggy skin as well as decreasing the appearance of different age spots. It also works as a protective oxidant, warding off free radicals that are often the cause of premature aging as well as other degenerative skin diseases. Unlike other oils, it helps maintain the body's natural antioxidant reserves as well as protects our skin from harmful ultraviolet rays which can further increase wrinkle formation.

3. Improves Athletic Performance – It can serve as source of quick energy during training. At the same time, it helps improve an athlete's endurance as well as keep their energy levels up through natural means.

4. Bones – It aids the body in the absorption of different nutrients such as magnesium and calcium, both of which are needed by the body to develop strong bones as well as prevent osteoporosis.

5. Diabetes – Virgin coconut oil can help when it comes to controlling blood sugar levels as well as in improving the body's ability to produce insulin. It can also help prevent and treat diabetes by enabling the body to utilize the blood glucose more efficiently. It can also provide ketones as an alternative source of energy and at the same time, effectively reduces the symptoms of diabetes along with lowering a person's risks of developing it.

6. Digestion – Improves the functions of our digestive system and helps prevent various stomach related problems which also includes IBS. It contains antimicrobial properties which can effectively fight off fungi, bacteria and parasites. All of which can cause serious indigestion. When it comes to mineral and nutrient absorption, it also makes the body more efficient and capable of taking the important stuff from the food that we eat. These also help if you're on a diet and trying to lose weight.

7. Hair Care – If used regularly on the hair, virgin coconut oil helps in making it grow healthier and shinier. It can also help in controlling dandruff as well as lice and lice eggs. If your hair has been significantly damaged by various treatments and you want it to go back to a much healthier state, regular application would hasten the regrowth and get rid

of damaged parts. Along with that, it can also greatly nourish your hair with the nutrients it needs, thus making for a great all natural conditioner.

8. Heart Health – If you're worried about its effects on your heart then fret not because it actually contains "good fat" that will not accumulate in your arteries and clog them up. It will not raise your LDL unlike other vegetable oils would. In fact, it is comprised of 50% lauric acid which can actually help in lowering high blood pressure as well as high cholesterol levels. In some cases, it has even reduced the risk of heart disease in people as well as prevented atherosclerosis.

9. Immune System – Virgin coconut oil contains lauric acid, antimicrobial lipids, caprylic acid as well as capric acid. These also have antibacterial, antifungal and antiviral properties that help in strengthening our immune systems. By taking it, you can also lower your risk of getting viral and bacterial infection, avoid influenza as well as be a bit more immune to cytomegalovirus and HIV. It also helps in treating and fighting off fungi and yeast which can cause ringworm problems, candidiasis, thrush, diaper rash and athlete's foot.

10. Kidney and Liver – When it comes to the kidney, not only will it aid in dissolving kidney stones, it can also help you prevent any related diseases. As for the liver, because of the MCFTA's contained in the virgin coconut oil, the liver needs to work less into converting it into energy therefore there isn't much strain on the organ itself.

11. Skin Care – Virgin coconut oil has a plethora of benefits when it comes to skin care. The first of which would be its ability to aid in the natural pH balance of the skin and helps in relieving any dryness or flaking brought on by an imbalance or dry weather. If you have oily skin, it is likely that you have a hard time looking for the right moisturizer for your skin. Look no further because coconut oil has the right elements for this purpose. It won't leave your skin feeling greasy. Besides those, it can also help in reducing the symptoms of eczema, psoriasis, dermatitis as well as a number of other skin problems.

More on Skin care

Other than just knowing the effects of virgin coconut oil on our skin, let's have an in-depth discussion regarding the connection of these two. We'll provide an explanation as to why this is happening. Additionally, we will introduce to you the other effects of using virgin coconut oil in your skin.

Hair Care

Skin is a large part of our body; after all, it covers each area and protects our internal organs from being exposed. This includes the scalp and our hair. The latter may be a non-living part of our body, but it is still made of cells.

Essential Oils Box Set #30: Coconut Oil for Easy Weight Loss & The Beginners Guide to Medical Plants

If you want a natural ingredient that can be used to care for your scalp and hair, virgin coconut oil is the right one to do the job. As mentioned, it is known as a moisturizing agent. Thus, it is the best cure for people who experience dry scalp or dandruff. It can even be used as a cure by those who have lice and lice eggs in their scalp. To use it, apply a small amount of virgin coconut oil on the scalp and massage it. Allow it to sit on your scalp between 10 and 20 minutes. You can choose to rinse the oil immediately, or leave it overnight and shampoo your scalp the next day.

Another benefit that your hair can get out of using coconut oil is that it can help you provide nourishment to your hair, and even help restore those who have dry and damaged hair. This is possible because the use of coconut oil helps prevent the loss of protein in the hair, which then contributes to undesirable hair conditions. Compared to other oils, coconut oil is more effective because one component that it has (which is the lauric acid) is able to penetrate the hair shaft and protect each strand from losing protein. Although most people believe that sunflower oil produces the same effect (since it contains linoleic acid, a triglyceride like lauric acid), research shows that linoleic is not able to penetrate the hair and prevent protein loss. It can be used to get rid of frizz, tangles, and dry split ends by applying a small amount of coconut oil on the affected area. With continued use, many people testify that it can make your hair manageable, shinier, and with increased body.

Taking care of skin problems

Aside from taking care of your crown, it is also used to get rid of several skin problems that you could have. The following are some of the conditions that can be alleviated with the use of virgin coconut oil:

- Aside from the skin problems that can be cured by coconut oil, another problem that can be overcame with its use is acne. This is because coconut oil is known for its anti-fungal and anti-bacterial properties, along with moisturizing the skin. Combined with medications prescribed by doctor (or even used on its own), you can experience positive results faster. The same anti-bacterial property is also useful in curing yeast infections. However, it is recommended that you consult with the doctor so that he/she can check if any of the lotions that you're using will produce a reaction when combined with coconut oil.

- If you experience scaling or cracking on the skin of your feet (which can either be a simple dry skin or athlete's foot), you can get rid of it with the use of coconut oil. If it is simple dry skin, it is cured because of the moisturizing effect of the oil. For athlete's foot, the anti-fungal property present in it acts to solve the problem. Used with other anti-fungal ingredients such as oregano and tea tree oil, your athlete's foot will be cured faster. This same moisturizing property can also be used even if your skin is not damaged. In most cases, it can replace commercial lotions that promise to hydrate and moisturize your skin.

- It can prevent and cure sunburn – rather than use an artificial sun block lotion, coconut oil can serve as a natural sun block. When it is applied, the heat that is supposed to cause the sunburn is filtered. On the other hand, if you already have sunburn, it can also be used to cure it. Because of the healing property that is present in it, using coconut oil can take away the discomfort caused by too much exposure from the sun. However, when using it as a cure, you need to make sure that the heat inside your body is already gone before you start applying it. By doing so, you can avoid trapping the heat inside your body. In most cases, you will need to wait for at least 24 to 72 hours before you can start with the treatment.

- Diaper rash, bruises, and bee stings can also be soothed with the use of virgin coconut oil. Because of the natural pH content, there is a significantly lower chance that the body will produce an allergic reaction when it is applied. But for you to be sure that your skin is not really allergic to it (especially if it is your first time to apply it on your skin), make a patch test first. This is done by applying a small amount of the oil on a small part of your skin. If there are no allergies, you can then apply it to the rest of your body.

- If you want to have an ageless skin and get rid of age spots, you can also apply coconut oil on the affected area; after all, it is also an anti-oxidant.

- Itching due to exposure to elements that may trigger it such as poison ivy or having chicken pox can be eased when the affected areas are applied with small amounts of coconut oil.

Hygiene and relaxation

Aside from being the cure to many skin problems, it can also be used for hygiene and relaxation such as the following:

- It can be used as a natural cleanser for any part of your body – even the face! Do you know that our body rids itself of grime or dirt with the use of oil that is called sebum? When you use coconut oil, it can act as an "artificial" sebum that will remove the dirt that your body has accumulated throughout the day!

- Just as how coconut oil can be used to remove dirt, it can also be used to easily remove make-up, especially oil-based ones such as mascara. This will help unclog the pores in your face. It can also serve as your lip balm, and get rid of cracks on your lips due to wind burn or use of lipstick.

- Due to the anti-bacterial quality of coconut oil, it can also be used as a deodorant. After all, the bacteria that accumulates on the skin folds such as the armpit is what causes the undesirable odor. To make your natural deodorant, you will need to mix coconut oil, baking soda, and cornstarch. For a more fragrant deodorant, you can include a small amount of your preferred scent on the mixture.

- It can be used as massage oil. Move away from the conventional baby oil, which is sticky and is not really absorbed by the skin. Aside from that, using coconut oil can also soothe sore and tired muscles. Just like the DIY deodorant, you can add a small amount of your preferred essential oil for a more soothing and fragrant massage experience.

- For a facial scrub and exfoliator of dead skin cells and white/blackheads, coconut oil can also be used. This is done by mixing the coconut oil with baking soda, oatmeal, and cinnamon or sugar.

- For men, coconut oil can also be used as a shaving and after-shave cream. Not only will it make your shaving experience faster (serving as a lubricant), it also promotes healing if ever you had wounds while shaving.

Nature has provided a healthy ingredient that can be used to make your skin healthier. Of course, it is also cheap. Just imagine how much you can save when you start using virgin coconut oil instead of all the artificial creams that contain toxic chemicals.

Virgin coconut oil and your oral health

Aside from the benefits that can be gained when applying coconut oil on your skin, its use is also said to give great benefits to your oral health. This section will discuss just how this oil can help your teeth and mouth to become healthy.

How is this possible?

As mentioned, coconut oil contains anti-bacterial and anti-fungal properties. These properties however, are not just effective in getting rid of wounds outside. It can still work wonders even inside your mouth, which is considered to be a host to a lot of bacteria.

These qualities make it effective in promoting your oral health. If the use of coconut oil is done alongside brushing and flossing your teeth, you are giving it better protection against the thriving of bacteria. It also protects the enamel of your teeth, making it stronger and prevents it from falling or getting extracted.

Another way how coconut oil can help improve your dental health is that it helps your body to easily absorb magnesium and calcium – two minerals that are important in strengthening your bones and teeth. This benefit can be achieved regardless of its application (whether applied topically or as an ingredient of your food).

Oil pulling

One practice that takes advantage of the abovementioned benefits that coconut oil has on your dental health is oil pulling. This practice has been adapted by the people of India for almost a thousand years, and is regaining popularity.

In this practice, the virgin coconut oil is believed to be the best mouthwash – not only is it natural and does not contain any toxic chemicals, it is also far effective in cleansing the mouth and removing any leftovers in-between teeth. It also removes bacteria that may cause various periodontal diseases such as gingivitis or gum recession. Additionally, it is said to give a great massage for the gums.

The procedure is easy. You will just need to use the coconut oil as a mouthwash and let it stay in your mouth for at least 15 minutes. Continuously swish your mouth so that the oil can reach every area inside. After 15 minutes, expel the mouthwash and proceed with brushing your teeth. Since you are using oil, the food debris will literally be pulled out of their hiding places.

Oil pulling is basically done during your shower time, as it gives you something else to do while gargling away the food debris and bacteria inside your mouth. However, make sure that you will never swallow the oil that was used for gargling; after all, you would not want to ingest the bacteria that you're trying to get out of your mouth.

Dental products using virgin coconut oil

Aside from using coconut oil as a mouthwash, it can also be used to make other products to improve your oral health.

- You can make your own toothpaste using coconut oil – without all the preservatives, chemicals, and sweeteners found on commercial toothpaste. This is done by mixing 1 part of baking soda with 1 part of coconut oil. For a "mint" taste, add a few drops of peppermint oil.

- It can also be used to get rid of other conditions related to your mouth. One of the most common oral problems that can be solved with its use is toothache. This is done by ingesting coconut oil mixed with clove oil. The anti-bacterial properties of the former and the analgesic (pain killing) property of the latter make it the best cure for toothache.

- Virgin coconut oil can also be used to as a cure for sore throat. This is done by taking in a spoonful of oil and allow it to roll slowly through your mouth (you will not swallow it intentionally). By doing so, you are allowing the oil to coat your throat and protect it. You also gain the benefit of fighting the infection that caused the sore throat.

Now that you have discovered the numerous health benefits that the use of coconut oil can bring, it would be easier for you to change your mind as to why you should include it in your diet as well as in your daily activities.

Chapter 7: Virgin Coconut Oil Diet Recipes

Alright, now that you know all about the different benefits that you can get from adding virgin coconut oil to your diet, you must be wondering about how you can do just that. If you're not too keen on taking the product directly, here are a few delicious ways through which you can add it to your daily menu.

Refreshing Smoothie Recipes:

I. Berry Coconut Smoothie

This smoothie is significantly high in antioxidant amounts and is one of the best when it comes to mixing with coconut oil. The flavors work very well together to create a refreshing and sweet taste. Because of the high antioxidant content, it is recommended that you have it as a dessert after a meal or before bed. It will efficiently cleanse your body.

Ingredients: 1 tablespoon of raw virgin coconut oil. 1 cup of unsweetened almond milk or one that's vanilla flavored. A cup of strawberries, you can also mix it with other varieties such as blueberries or raspberries. 5 ice cubes. You can also add in a scoop of your favorite protein shake if you intend to turn it into a meal smoothie.

To make: Simply blend together and serve chilled.

II. Island Dream Smoothie

This smoothie features spirulina, a protein-rich superfood. It has a rich, brilliant green color and by adding some stevia into it, a refreshing sweetness that also masks the earthy taste brought by the spirulina. If you're on a diet and still looking for something healthy to eat, this would be the best option to try. It contains many of the nutrients that your body needs for the day without the added calories!

Ingredients: A cup of coconut water (or a regular one, it depends on what you like). 1 to 2 tablespoons of raw virgin coconut oil depending on what you need. A tablespoon of organic spirulina powder mixed with half a cup of frozen banana and pineapples. A packet of NuNaturals Stevia or another brand that you prefer. A handful of spinach and at least 5 ice cubes.

To make: Simply blend and serve chilled.

III. Superfood Smoothie

On the subject of superfoods, here's one that many weight watchers would certainly enjoy. This smoothie recipe contains 5 different superfoods that are needed on a daily basis when it comes to energy, hormonal balance, skin and metabolism. They are also significantly high when it comes to raw amino acids and would make for a great meal replacement, as a snack or even as an afternoon pick me up. It would make you feel full and energized but without the added calories and fats!

Ingredients: A cup of unsweetened vanilla coconut milk or almond milk depending on your tastes. ¼ cup of frozen blueberries. A teaspoon of maca powder and raw cacao powder as well as a teaspoon of your favorite green powder; doesn't matter which brand. 1 scoop of protein powder, use your favorite! 1 teaspoon of acai powder or goji powder if that's something you like more. 1 teaspoon of vanilla extract, make sure it's gluten free. 2 tablespoons of virgin coconut oil and add a handful of spinach. Lastly, 5 to 6 pieces ice cubes.

To make: Blend, chill and serve.

IV. Coconut Acai Smoothie

Acai, another well-known superfood makes an appearance in this delicious and very filling smoothie. It contains a lot of Omega 3 fatty acids, protein as well as a generous amount of antioxidants which is great for speeding up your metabolism and of course, hastening weight loss as well. If you air that with the different health benefits that virgin coconut oil can offer and you've got yourself a smoothie that could easily replace a meal. Have it as a snack or drink it for breakfast!

Ingredients: 1 cup of unsweetened coconut milk or almond milk. 1 frozen packet of acai pulp as well as 2 tablespoons of coconut oil. 1 packet of Stevia powder as well as a dash or vanilla or cinnamon for added sweetness and flavor.

To make: Simply blend and serve.

V. Coconut and Kale Smoothie

Kale and coconut may seem like an unlikely pair but they do make for a refreshing and filling green smoothie that could easily replace any of your meals for the day. It contains proteins as well as different vitamins, iron and fiber as well as Omega 3's. All of which are enough to power you through the day. You can have it from breakfast or as a dessert after one of your meals. It would make you feel as if you've just snacked on a really delicious salad.

Ingredients: 1 cup of unsweetened vanilla milk or coconut milk if this is more of your taste. You will also need 1 cup of kale, 1 cup of spinach as well as half a frozen banana. ¼ cup of frozen blueberries, 1 to 2 tablespoons of virgin coconut oil along with a dash of cinnamon. Lastly, add 5 ice cubes into the mix.

To make: Simply blend and chill before serving.

VI. Hot cocoa with virgin coconut oil

Essential Oils Box Set #30: Coconut Oil for Easy Weight Loss & The Beginners Guide to Medical Plants

Although technically not considered a smoothie, cocoa is a common beverage for many people. This version of hot cocoa however, integrates virgin coconut oil to give it a healthier twist.

Ingredients:

1 tablespoon of cocoa powder

1 tablespoon of virgin coconut oil

¼ teaspoon of organic sugar

A pinch of salt

Procedure:

1. Pour hot water on the mug and let it sit for at least 20 seconds. After this, empty the mug.

2. Using the emptied mug, pour the virgin coconut oil and the cocoa powder. The oil is used to dissolve the powder and make the mixture. Add the salt as well.

3. To get rid of the cocoa's bitter taste, use a small amount of organic sugar.

4. Add hot water on the concentrated cocoa mixture. To suit your taste, you can add milk and your preferred sweetener. However, keep in mind that you should use sweeteners minimally, even if it is organic.

Entrees:

I. Coconut Fried Shrimp

If you're looking to change up your meals to something much healthier and more appropriate when it comes to weight loss then this recipe is something you should try. Filling, delicious and low in calories, you're sure to enjoy it.

Ingredients: You will need a pound of peeled fresh shrimp. ½ cup of organic coconut flour. ¼ cup of organic cornstarch mixed with ½ a teaspoon of fine salt. You will also need ½ a cup of water, 2 eggs and ½ cups of organic shredded coconut. Add ½ cup of virgin coconut oil and ½ cup of virgin palm oil to the mix and you're done.

To make: Mix the starch, the coconut flour, salt, water and the eggs in a bowl. Using a fork, blend it all together until the starches get dissolved. Dip the shrimp in this simple batter before rolling it onto the shredded coconut. Heat your palm and coconut oils in a skillet at about 375 degrees then fry the shrimp until it becomes golden brown. A minute for each side should be enough because if you overcook shrimp, it can easily become a little rubbery in texture. To remove the excess oil, simply drain the shrimp on paper towels before you serve it. As an alternative to the palm oil, you can also make use of organic palm shortening instead.

II. Coconut Chicken Strips with Honey Mustard

Typically, fried chicken isn't something dieters would want to touch but with this recipe, you'll be able to enjoy this delicious food guilt free while getting to enjoy the benefits of consuming coconut oil as well. Here's what you need to do:

Ingredients: 1 ½ cups of coconut chips or shredded coconut depending on your preferences. 1 ½ pounds of organic chicken breasts that has been cut into strips, this is the healthiest part of the chicken. You will also need 2 tablespoons of butter, olive and virgin coconut oil. 1 tablespoon of flour mixed with 1 teaspoon of nutmeg. Lastly, you'll need ½ a cup of prepared mustard and 2 tablespoons of honey.

To make: To get started, turn your own on and set it to broil. Set your coconut shreds evenly on a baking sheet and toast this until it becomes slightly browned. Removed from the oven and let it cool to one side. Next, pre-heat your own to 375 degrees and while that's heating up, mix your flour, nutmeg and the toasted coconut into one bowl. Place your chicken strips in there and drizzle it with the coconut oil. You can skip using butter for this recipe if you don't like it. Prepare your cookie sheet by putting some of the coconut oil on it as well; this is so it doesn't end up sticking while it cooks. Coat your chicken evenly with the dry mixture before you bake it. Leave it baking for at least ten minutes or until it becomes thoroughly cooked. After, prepare the mustard and honey by simply mixing both together.

III. Mussels in Lemongrass Broth

For people whose cooking skills are quite advanced, you can try this complex but equally healthy appetizer.

Ingredients:

This dish needs two preparations; for the mussel soup and for the lemongrass stock. Obviously, their ingredients are different.

For the lemongrass stock:

6 cups of water (cold)

4 stalk of lemongrass; remove the dry outer leaves

8 slices of ginger (thin)

1 piece of sliced yellow onion

1 teaspoon of coriander seed

½ teaspoon of salt

For the mussel soup:

1 kilogram of mussels

3 tablespoons of olive oil

2 tablespoons of virgin coconut oil

1 ½ kilos of yellow-orange tomatoes; the core should be removed and sliced into 4 equal pieces

3 cloves of garlic; should be peeled and sliced

½ piece of a medium-sized onion; should be sliced thinly

6-8 pieces of Italian basil leaves

1 teaspoon of ginger; should be grated

Salt and ground pepper

1 liter of lemongrass stock

To make the recipe, you need to prepare the lemongrass stock first. This is done by first placing the lemongrass in a hard surface (such as a chopping board) and pounding it gently. Doing so will release its oils. After this, all the ingredients (including the pounded lemongrass) should be combined in the stockpot. Bring it to a boil, simmer, and cook without the pot cover for at least 40 minutes. Once you're done cooking, pour it through the strainer. Press the vegetables firmly so that all liquids will be drained before they are discarded.

After making the stock, you can now make the dish. This is done by following this procedure:

1. Start by heating 1 tablespoon of olive oil and the prepared amount of virgin coconut oil in medium heat using a soup pot.

2. Add the garlic, ginger, and onion; your cue to stop cooking is when the onion is translucent.

3. Add the tomatoes and cook for at least 5 minutes.

4. After this, you can now pour the lemongrass stock along with the basil leaves. Add salt and pepper depending on your taste preference. Let it simmer for at least 10 minutes.

5. Puree the mixture in a blender. While doing so, add the remaining amount of olive oil until the mixture is smooth. Add more salt if necessary.

6. Once you're done with the puree, return it to the pot. Let it simmer, add the mussels, and cover. Cook until the shells have opened; discard any mussel whose shells did not open. Serve.

Mussels and other shellfish are good sources of protein and sodium without packing in on calories. It also contains low saturated fat. This recipe is also healthier because of the vegetable stock that was used to make it. It is also appealing for pregnant mothers due to the folic acid (better known as folate) that it contains – a nutrient that can help reduce the risk of the baby to develop congenital malformations.

IV. Chicken Curry with Virgin Coconut Oil

If you want to adapt the habit of using virgin coconut oil in your diet, you need to learn how you can integrate it with dishes that you were already used to eating. One dish that is popular in many places all over the world is the curry. For this version of the chicken curry, we will introduce the use of virgin coconut oil.

Ingredients:

3 to 4 portions of chicken

½ tablespoon of curry powder

1 tablespoon of coconut flour

1 ½ tablespoon of virgin coconut oil

1 cup of chicken stock (this can be made using some of the unused parts of the chicken such as the neck)

1/8 cup of onions, chopped

2 cloves of garlic

¼ tablespoon of salt

½ tablespoon of fresh ginger root, chopped

1/4 cup of water

1/8 teaspoon of black pepper

Procedure:

To make the dish, these steps should be followed:

1. Sauté the ginger, garlic, and onion in a frying pan using coconut oil. After a few minutes, add the chicken. Cook until it is slightly brown.

2. Once the chicken is cooked, add the chicken stock and let it simmer for at least 15 minutes.

3. After the specified time, add the black pepper, salt, and curry powder, and cover the cooking pan. Cook for another 5 minutes.

4. Dissolve the coconut flour in water, and add it to the dish. Once added to the mixture, cook for 5 minutes then serve.

For this recipe, coconut milk was substituted with coconut flour dissolved in water. Virgin coconut oil was also used to fry and sauté the chicken, which contains less fat compared to other oils.

This can be a good alternative in your weekly food plan, as you won't get stuck on fish and beef or pork. Chicken allows you to eat meat and give your body the protein that it needs while taking in lower fat content.

V. Pan seared cod fillet with basil and garlic cream

The codfish (or cod for short) is an ingredient known for being a source of vitamin A, D, and E, and also a source of omega 3 fatty acids (which is good for the heart). The benefits of this ingredient will further be augmented with the use of virgin coconut oil.

Ingredients:

450 grams of cod fillet

2 tablespoons of virgin coconut oil

1 slice of lime

Salt and fresh ground pepper

For making the cream, you will need the following:

¼ cup of finely chopped basil leaves

3 cloves of minced garlic

1 ½ ounce of soft goat cheese

1/3 cup of grated parmesan cheese

¼ cup of sour cream

Procedure:

1. Start by seasoning the cod on all sides with salt and pepper. Set aside and prepare the cream.

2. The cream is made by mixing the goat cheese to break its large clumps. After this, you will add the basil, garlic, and the remaining ingredients. Mix thoroughly. You can add the desired amount of sour cream to adjust the taste to your liking. Set this aside.

3. Heat the coconut oil in high heat using a large skillet. Once the oil is heated, sear the cod fillets for around 8 to 10 minutes in medium heat, turning it over once. After the fillet was turned over, squeeze the lime juice over the fillet before you resume with cooking. The cod is cooked once it's slightly browned.

4. Serve by adding lime juice or a lime wedge, and use a generous amount of the cream as its topping.

Most people sear their dishes using butter along with the coconut oil for improved taste. For this recipe however, the use of the butter was totally replaced with an additional amount of coconut oil; from 1 tablespoon of virgin coconut oil and butter separately, it was changed to 2 tablespoons of oil and eliminated the butter.

VI. Sautéed vegetables and beef

Most kids prefer beef over vegetables nowadays. It is only when they're combined that they are enticed to eat a vegetable dish. Take this opportunity to introduce virgin coconut oil in their diet and system by using it to cook this dish.

Ingredients:

450 grams of lean beef; should be sliced thinly

½ cup of beef broth

4 tablespoons of virgin coconut oil

2 tablespoons of soy sauce

2 tablespoons of sherry

1 cup of green peas; each piece should be cut into 1 inch

1 cup of sliced mushrooms

1 cup of bean sprouts

1 teaspoon of ginger root; should be sliced thinly

1 medium-sized carrot sliced thinly

½ cup of green onions, with each piece cut into 1 inch

A pinch of organic sugar

Salt

Procedure:

1. Start by heating the virgin coconut oil in a pan. Once heated, use it to fry the beef until it is browned. After frying, remove the beef from the pan and drain its oil.

2. Stir fry the onion and ginger using 2 tablespoons of virgin coconut oil for at least 1 minute.

3. Once you're done with stir frying, add the beef broth and stir.

4. Let the mixture simmer for at least 2 minutes. After this, add the soy sauce, sherry, and organic sugar.

5. Add the beans and bean sprouts, carrots, and mushrooms. Continue stirring until the vegetables are crisp. Add salt to match your taste preference. Serve while hot.

Desserts

I. Peanut Butter Granola With Coconut Oil

If you're looking for something sweet yet healthy to satisfy your sweet tooth then this recipe would surely whet your appetite.

Ingredients: 1/3 cup of raw honey as well as ½ cup of peanut butter. You will also need a tablespoon of coconut cream and ¼ cup of coconut oil. Add 2 cups of oatmeal to that along with ¾ cup of coconut flakes.

To make: Making this dessert snack is actually pretty simple and would take very little time. To get started, preheat your oven to 275 degrees. Then, mix all of your ingredients together, except for the coconut and oatmeal, in a saucepan. Make sure that you keep it at a very low heat. Mix this until it becomes smooth. Once the consistency is to your liking, simply add the oatmeal and coconut flakes. Stir these in well. Spread the mixture onto an oiled cookie sheet and put it in the preheated oven for at least 10 minutes. Stir it once more and get the air bubbles to pop before putting it back in for another 10 minutes. Once done, let it cool before serving. This recipe is best eaten with milk and would be great snacks between your meals whenever you're craving.

II. Gluten-free Zucchini Pancakes

Looking for a refreshing lunch or something to snack on in-between your meals? This recipe would certainly fit great into that need.

Ingredients: 1 medium stalk zucchini; make sure that the ends have been removed and have it coarsely grated. You will also need 2 eggs, 2 to 3 tablespoons of virgin coconut oil as well as a teaspoon of red onion that's been finely chopped. Freshly ground black pepper, 2 teaspoons of asiago cheese that's been grated, this would add flavor to the meal. 2 to 3 basil leaves, finely minced. Lastly, you will also need a teaspoon of coconut flour and a dash of salt to taste.

To make: In a bowl, add your grated zucchini and eggs together, mix it thoroughly and make sure everything is coated. Heat your coconut oil in a large skillet then add black pepper, onion, asiago cheese, and some basil to your zucchini. If the mixture is a little too liquid for your liking, add a few dashes of the coconut oil to thicken it. When the oil is hot enough, carefully fork some of the batter into the pan and then mash it down to spread it. Make sure that you do this evenly so you make pancakes that aren't too thin. Let each side cook for about a minute or two, or up until it becomes a deeper brown shade. Once completely cooked, drain the excess oil on paper towels before serving.

III.Gluten-free Blackberry Banana Muffin

If you are allergic to gluten but loves to eat baked goods, then this recipe is for you.

Ingredients:

8 eggs

2 bananas; should be ripe and mashed

5 tablespoons of maple syrup

3 teaspoons of cinnamon

2 teaspoons of vanilla extract

1 teaspoon of baking powder

1 cup of blackberries

¾ cup of coconut flour

½ cup of virgin coconut oil

½ teaspoon of salt

Procedure:

1. Start by pre-heating your oven to at least 177 degrees Celsius.

2. Combine all the ingredients in a mixing bowl except for the baking powder and coconut flour.

3. Mix the contents of the bowl up to medium speed until everything is blended well.

4. Add the baking powder and coconut flour, and resume with mixing. Make sure that the mixture is combined smoothly.

5. Pour the mixture on muffin tins. Make sure that the inside is greased to avoid sticking. Bake for at least 20 to 25 minutes, or until the food is firm when touched.

This recipe went away with the use of the conventional flour (which is made of wheat, the source of gluten). Instead, it used coconut flour. This recipe also used two nutritious fruits – namely, banana and blackberry. Banana aids in digestion, contains fiber, and is a good source of potassium. Blackberry, on the other hand, is an excellent source of antioxidants, which lowers the risk of developing diseases. It can also contribute to the cell's regeneration, making it a good food for those who want to look younger than their actual age.

IV. Fruit tart – without baking

All of us know that tart is another baked good. But do you know that you can make one even without baking? What's better is that it's healthy and uses virgin coconut oil! This is an easy to prepare and no-bake version of fruit tart.

Ingredients:

For this recipe, you will need three sets of ingredients – crust, custard, and toppings.

For the crust:

1/8 cup of dried coconut

¼ cup of pitted dates

1 cup of raw macadamia nuts (if not available, you can also use pecans or walnuts)

For the custard:

2 cups of chopped cashews; should soaked for at least 30 minutes

½ cup virgin coconut oil

½ cup of raw honey

½ cup of lime juice

1 teaspoon of vanilla

1 teaspoon of salt

The toppings would be your preferred fruit(s).

Procedure:

1. To prepare the crust, you must use the food processor to process the dates and nuts. Once the crust was made, place it on a tart pan. Sprinkle the dried coconut on the pan; this will prevent the crust from sticking into the pan.

2. For the custard, you will have to blend the cashews, slightly warm coconut oil (should never be microwaved), honey, lime, vanilla, and salt. Blend until the custard is smooth and suits your taste.

3. Pour the custard in the crust. Make sure that there are no air bubbles. This is done by tapping the tart pan on the table.

4. Place the pan in the freezer until it is slightly firm. Once your tart is such, temporarily remove from the freezer to decorate it using your preferred fruits.

5. After placing the toppings, place it back in the freezer for around 10 to 20 minutes. This will make the tart firm. Serve after the specified time for freezing.

This recipe also did not use wheat to make the crust. Instead, it used whole grains (dates), which are good sources of fiber. The nuts are also sources of fats that are good for the heart, and the fresh fruits used as toppings are good sources of nutrients.

Keep your body healthy and looking great by substituting the conventional oils that you use for cooking with virgin coconut oil. By doing so, you will be taking one step closer towards a better health and life.

Chapter 8: Complement Your Virgin Coconut Oil Regimen

So there you have it, a step by step guide to learning more about virgin coconut oil and its many different uses, including how it can help you lose weight. Remember, it's important to learn the basics before you get started as there is a difference between regular coconut oil and the virgin variety. As you have learned, the latter is healthier and supports many of the health benefits that your body needs, especially if you're trying to lose weight and changing up your diet.

Keep these in mind:

To lose weight using virgin coconut oil, it doesn't necessarily mean that you simply have to consume it and wait for the results. It would still require a bit of work.

1. Change your diet into something healthier and incorporate virgin coconut oil into your daily menu using some of the recipes provided above. Be disciplined, however, and avoid overindulging. But because coconut oil would help you feel fuller for longer, snacking can be easily avoided.

2. Aside from taking it easy on the entrees, you should also control yourself from overindulging on desserts that contains virgin coconut oil. Just because they contain healthy fat and other nutrients that you can consume more than what you're supposed to. Most desserts are still sweet, which should be limited if you want to have a healthier body. Remember that getting your desired body revolves around control of what and how much you eat.

3. If possible, integrate other forms of coconut in your food plan. Do not be limited to using virgin coconut oil only. As you will notice from some of the recipes on the previous chapter, other coconut-related products are used. One example would be the coconut flour. Since it is also derived from the same source, it is safe to assume that the product also contains the components that can be found in virgin coconut oil.

4. Aside from the use of coconut oil, it is also recommended that you use fresh or organic ingredients when cooking your dishes. Virgin coconut oil alone cannot do the job of keeping you healthy if everything else that you ingest is not good for the body.

5. Get your kids used to consuming virgin coconut oil by integrating in the food that you prepare. By doing so, you can reduce their risk of getting childhood obesity. Additionally, introduce to them the topical use of virgin coconut oil. Use it as your sunblock during summer, or use it as their shampoo. This will make them further appreciate what virgin coconut oil can do for them.

6. Do exercise. Simply eating virgin coconut oil is not enough to do the trick. Add a regular exercise routine to your everyday tasks. It doesn't have to be tedious but you will need to sweat and use your muscles for it. Brisk walking, yoga, or something as simple as going up and down the first two steps of the stairs would be good enough as long as you do it every day.

7. Keep a steady supply of virgin coconut oil in the house. In order to integrate virgin coconut oil into one's diet, it is important that a bottle or jar of it is always within reach. Keep a bottle of it in your office desk, in your room, in the kitchen and even in the bathroom! This will be a constant reminder to use it as much as possible, whenever needed. Remember that aside from being a weight loss aid, it is also excellent for skin and hair care, so keep it handy.

8. Shop in your local farmer's market. As much as possible, purchase from local farmers instead of buying fresh produce in grocery stores. Local farmers usually sell fresh vegetables and fruits without the use of commercial grade pesticides. They also sell free range meat products which is free from hormones and other chemicals.

9. Lastly, make the necessary lifestyle changes. There are certain habits that we have which can hinder weight loss. Look at your habits, cross out the bad ones and simply change them into something better.

Conclusion

Thank you again for purchasing this book!

I hope this book was able to help you to better understand how virgin coconut oil benefits our health and body, as well as how it can help dieters achieve their weight loss goals without compromising their good health.

The next step is to apply all that you have learned in this eBook and watch the transformation happen on you.

Finally, if you enjoyed this book, please take the time to share your thoughts and post a review on Amazon. We do our best to reach out to readers and provide the best value we can. Your positive review will help us achieve that. It'd be greatly appreciated!

Thank you and good luck!

Book 2

The Beginners Guide to Medicinal Plants

BY LINDSEY P

Everything You Need to Know About the Healing Properties of Plants & Herbs, How to Grow and Harvest Them

Essential Oils Box Set #30: Coconut Oil for Easy Weight Loss & The Beginners Guide to Medical Plants

Table Of Contents

Introduction

I want to thank you and congratulate you for purchasing the book, *"The Beginners Guide to Medicinal Plants"*.

This book contains proven steps and strategies on how to successfully grow medicinal plants and herbs right at the very comfort of your own home.

Featured in this book are some of the most common mistakes when putting up a medicinal garden at home and how to avoid committing such mistakes. Also featured in this book are some of the best types of medicinal plants to grow at home.

Thanks again for purchasing this book, I hope you enjoy it!

Chapter 1: Guide to Growing a Medicinal Herb Garden

Growing medicinal plants and herbs indoor is a popular hobby for a lot of gardeners. One of the greatest reasons to plant medicinal plants indoor is to have a ready supply of these beneficial herbs. These herbs are those that you commonly snip into your sauces and soups. They can also be used to soothe an itchy rash or cough. Growing medicinal herbs may not sound to be very appealing, however you can benefit from growing these plants that can provide instant relief for many illnesses that can happen anytime of the day.

It would also be wonderful to be able to cut a sprig of thyme while boiling water and prepare a fresh cup of thyme tea that is fragrant and vibrant. Since it is fresh, you'll sure it is effective since it's fresh.

So what kind of medicinal plants should you grow? The next chapter of this book features a list of different herbs and medicinal plants that you can grow at home. The list is just a good starting point for easy to find and easy to grow herbs. The same plants that you can use in cooking daily may also be used as teas, salves, washes and tinctures. You can also make cough syrup and cough drops with the very same herbal plants that you grow in the comforts of your own home.

No matter how you thoroughly care for your medicinal plants, in the long run, they will have to be replaced. If this should happen during the colder days, you will have to take into account the growing time, before they will be big enough for harvest. Commonly, this will take about 4 to 6 weeks. You can make use of these herbs not only for cooking but for medicinal purposes as well.

What problems can you possibly encounter while growing medicinal plants and herbs in your home garden? While herbs typically suffer from much less issues that flowers and vegetables do, there are a few things that should be looked out for. Plants grown in your home garden may also encounter some basic problems such as molds or mildew problems, insect damage and most of all, fertilizer issues. To remedy these problems, you must know the following guidelines:

1. Home Garden Temperature

   While most of us think our homes as a temperate area would be ideal for growing plants, this is not always the case.

   A plant requires light in order to make food, a process which we know as photosynthesis. While plants are very adaptable, they grow best within a 70 to 75 degree range. A plant utilizes more energy when the temperature is warm than when it is cold. Plants can adapt to a cooler room, for instance, with an air conditioner. The plants will begin the process of photosynthesis with the increase in temperature and there will be no sunlight to produce food. When this happens, the plants will not most likely to thrive and will probably die.

So what is the best temperature for growing medicinal herbs?

Plants grow best when there is at least a 10 degree fall in temperature during the night. During the summer, the temperature tends to get high and stay high. Plants get stressed and become highly susceptible to diseases. They grow less and can drop leaves, weaken and die, despite sufficient watering. If you are growing herbs indoors, it would be a good idea to grow them around a room based on available temperature zones. Save a lot of money and be stress-free by working on with what you already have instead of trying to make big modifications that work against the natural rhythm of your home environment.

2. Home Garden Fertilizer

Once you have already decided on which type of herbs that you will grow in your home garden, you will now have to choose the most suitable fertilizer for them. Not all fertilizers are created the same. While most have advertising claims, these fertilizers may be overused enough to damage your medicinal herbs grown at home.

What kinds of fertilizers can be used at home? There are a lot of fertilizer types that will work for your medicinal herb garden at home. For indoor plants, you can try using a variety that can be dissolved in water (water-soluble). This particular type of fertilizer may come in packaged granular form that you measure and dissolve in water prior to application. It may also come in the form of a fish emulsion, which is a concentrated variety and is combined with water before application.

Regardless on the type of fertilizer that you choose to use, you must apply it at one quarter of the packaging's recommended amount. Apply this light mixture once every week. For a more effective application, make sure to water your plants thoroughly and then apply the prepared fertilizer solution. This technique will allow for better absorption by the plant.

More importantly, make sure that you do a monthly flushing of your medicinal plants. This can be done by placing the plant in a sink and water entirely, allowing the excess water to draw off. Once the dripping stops, water completely once again. This technique will get rid of any salts that may have accumulated in the plant's soil.

Chapter 2: Easy Guide to Successfully Grow Herbs and Medicinal Plants at Home

Follow this easy step-by-step guide to start with your medicinal herb garden at home:

1. Choose your herbs. When growing medicinal herbs at home, it is important to have a good variety of herbs as well as companion plants. Some of the good choice include the following:

   - Hot pepper

   - Strawberries

   - Oregano

   - Thyme

   - Lime basil

   - Mint

   - Common basil

   - Sage

   - Lemon balm

   - Sweet marjoram

2. Prepare your pot. Be sure that the pots that you will be using for your medicinal plants have holes at the bottom to provide good drainage. With a grit or gravel, pour to about a quarter of the pot's depth. This will allow the water to steep out from the soil's bottom.

3. Fill. When the gravel is already in place, begin to fill the pot with soil-based or multi-purpose compost. Fill t about three (3) quarters of the pot's remaining space.

4. Begin planting – put the medicinal plants into the pot, with around 15 centimeters between each stem. Squeeze every plant lightly from its temporary pot. To encourage the plants to spread out, tease the roots from the root ball.

5. Put the trailing plants near the edge and the taller ones in the center of the display. This technique will endure the best growth for your plants. DO not worry if the display may seem to appear messy at first. This will begin to fill out and look lush in just a few weeks.

6. Fill in the spaces around the plants. When you are already satisfied with the positions, begin filling in the gaps in between the plants with compost. Tightly push the compost into the spaces by pushing your fingers deep into the soil. Be careful not to injure the roots. Add more if needed. To avoid overflowing when being waters, leave a few centimeters between the rim of the pot and the soil.

7. Top the plants. Cut the taller plants' top. This will encourage them to bush out and give more fresh leaves to pick during harvest time.

8. Fertilize regularly. Purchase a controlled release fertilizer which should last a whole season. This will mean that you won't have to feed the pot again.

9. Water. Water your plants thoroughly or until the water begins to drain out of the pot's bottom. Medicinal plants usually like to dry out between watering and some types of medicinal plants such as Rosemary can easily be over-watered.

Growing herbs and medicinal plants at home is an easy yet a very rewarding hobby. Below are seven (7) key steps that will surely help you to successfully grow a healthy medicinal herb at home:

1. Keep an eye on Pests

   Medicinal herbs are generally not bothered so much about pests as much as flowers and vegetables can be. In an indoor garden however, the non-natural conditions may increase the possibility of a pest problem. To keep pests from damaging your medicinal plants in your indoor garden, make sure to keep a close eye. At the very first sight of infestation, make use of a soapy spray. You may also handpick any pests that you may have come to notices and put sticky traps to get rid of the rest.

2. Water your plants regularly

   Medicinal herbs require thorough attention when it comes to watering. Whether your medicinal plants likes drier conditions or extra moisture, it is never a good idea to have plants to be sitting in water.

3. Apply fertilizer

   Always keep in mind that medicinal plants grown indoors require a special fertilization schedule than those which are planted in an outdoor environment.

4. Be mindful of the soil

Indoor gardening soil needs to have effective exceptional drainage. It also needs to be light. Whether your medicinal plants like drier conditions or with extra moisture, having your plants to sit in water is never a good idea. Specifically buy potting soil. You may also prepare your own by using a part of peat moss, a part of sand and a part of bagged potting soil.

5. Ensure proper circulation

Medicinal plants require sufficient airflow to keep pests and bacterial organisms at bay. Just make sure to keep the air moving in the area where you will grow your medicinal plants.

6. Check your temperature

Keep your planting area at constant temperature. The ideal temperature for a home garden is about 60 to 70 degrees.

7. Provide enough light

Provide about 14 to 16 hours of artificial light to keep your medicinal plants healthy. You can also alternatively expose them to natural light for about 6 hours a day.

Chapter 3: The Best Medicinal Plants to Grow at Home

Do you have a small space at home to grow some plants? Why not grow some medicinal plants? Growing your own medicinal plants will not only get a lot of enjoyment but this will also provide medicinal relief at the comforts of your own home. While herbal remedies must never take the place of professional health care, it would be nice to have a sense of self-help should you ever end up having to need instant relief. Below is a list of the best plants to start your own personal medicinal plants garden:

1. Echinacea – this herb is also popularly known as the purple coneflower. Echinacea is an American perennial wildflower which is popularly known for its stimulating effects in the immune system. Preparations made with this wonder herb are used for the treatment of flu, colds, minor infections and a wide range of various illnesses.

2. Lavender – is medicinal plant which is commonly used as a fragrance these days. Lavender has been widely used since ancient times to reduce swelling, provide relief for rashes and itching and to treat burns, bug bites and other skin orders.

3. Lemon Balm – Prepare potent lemonade by adding bruised lemon balm leaves into your drink. This herb is commonly used as a calming "night tea" to combat insomnia. It can also make an effective topical relief for cold sores.

4. Comfrey – The roots of this wonder herb are cooked and mashed to make a potent topical relief for sprains, burns, bruises and arthritis. Just do not eat it. There is a study which reported that this herb can potentially damage the liver in eaten in significant amounts.

5. St. John's Wort – this wonder herb can lift the mood very well that you must keep from using this when you are already taking other forms of anti-depressants. The flowers and leaves of this herb may be used to prepare a tea. They can also be soaked in liquor to make a tincture. In a recent announcement, the FDA warned the public that there was a risk of adverse reactions between this herb and certain prescription drugs used for the treatment of cancer, transplant rejection, heart disease and AIDS, among others.

6. Borage – this potent herb has beautiful flowers that may be soaked in alcohol to prepare a powerful tonic that can boost your mood. The flowers and leaves may be used in tea preparations, eaten raw or soaked in liquor or wine to flavor the drink. The fresh plant provides a salty flavor with a cucumber-like smell.

7. Peppermint – this medicinal plant can be an effective tonic to promote better digestion. However, peppermint and any other strong mints such as pennyroyal must not be taken by women who are pregnant or possibly be pregnant. Drinks and foods that have fresh strong mint leaf can be harmful to the baby.

8. Pennyroyal – just like peppermint, pennyroyal is a great smelling mint which can be crushed and topically applied to the skin as a very powerful insect repellent. The leaves of pennyroyal can be crushed and topically applied to wounds as an antiseptic agent. It can also be used in tea preparations to tame upset stomach, however, do not over do it. The maximum recommendation is 2 cups daily. Consuming more than this recommendation may cause cramps and nausea.

9. Aloe vera – is a plant native to tropical Africa. This plant has spread worldwide as a first medicinal herb that provides soothing effects for scalds and burns. Aloe vera is best grown in a container so that it can be easily transferred indoors during the winter season.

10. Yarrow – for someone who's about to start a medicinal garden at home, yarrow is usually the top pick. This herb is a beautiful perennial plant that can serve a lot of different uses. Crushed yarrow flowers and leaves may be directly applied to scratches and cuts to reduce the chances of infections and to stop bleeding.

11. Slippery Elm – the inner back of this wonder herb can be ground and made into a nutrient-rich porridge-like soup. This can be an effective remedy for sore throat. In addition to this, the inner bark of this herb can be soothe irritations in the digestive tract.

12. Fenugreek – the seeds of this medicinal plant are nourishing and used to:

    • Restore a dull sense of taste

    • Freshen the breath

    • Ease labor pains

    • Ease painful menstruation

    • Help in insufficient lactation

    • Promote better digestion

    • Help for late onset diabetes

    • Darin off sweat ducts

    • Treat inflammation and ulcers of the intestines and stomach

- Reduce blood cholesterol levels

- Inhibit cancer of the liver

- Encourage weight gain

13. Feverfew – is a plant which can be made into tea for the treatment of fevers, colds and arthritis. This plant is said to have sedative properties. It can also regulate menstruation. A feverfew infusion may be used to bathe swollen feet. It can also be made into a tincture for the treatment of bruises. Chewing about 4 pieces of leaves daily has been proven to be an effective cure for some migraine headaches.

14. Comfrey – an herb which contains allantoin. This substance is a cell proliferant which boosts the natural replacement of body cells. Comfrey is widely known for its ability to build strong teeth and bones in children. Comfrey is safer to use externally than internally. This wonder herb is used to treat a wider variety of health issues including the following:

- Varicose veins

- Eczema

- Sores

- Sprains

- Bruises

- Cuts

- Acne

- Severe burns

- Varicose and gastric ulcers

- Arthritis

- Sprains

- Broken bones

- Bronchial problems

15. Milk Thistle – this powerful herb can protect and improve the function of the liver. This herb may be taken internally to help treat the following:

- The effects of a hangover

- The growth of cancer cells in prostate, cervical and breast cancer

- Insulin resistance in patients suffering from type 2 diabetes who also have cirrhosis

- Increased cholesterol levels

- Liver inflammation or hepatitis

- Jaundice

- Gall bladder diseases

- Liver diseases

16. Wu Wei Zi – the fruit of this herb are reported to stimulate the central nervous system when used in low doses. In large doses, the fruits are said to depress the central nervous system while regulating the cardiovascular system. The seeds of this herb are used in the treatment of cancer. When used externally, this herb is used to treat allergic and irritating skin problems. Internally, this herb is used to treat the following conditions:

- Diabetes

- Hepatitis

- Hyperacidity

- Poor memory

- Insomnia

- Palpitations

- Chronic diarrhea

- Involuntary ejaculation

- Urinary disorders

- Night sweats

- Asthma

- Dry coughs

17. Sage – the latin name for this herb, "salvia", means to heal. When used internally, this herb treats the following conditions:

- Menopausal problems

- Femal sterility

- Depression

- Anxiety

- Excessive salivation

- Excessive perspiration

- Excessive lactation

- Liver issues

- Flatulence

- Indigestion

When used externally, sage is used for:

  - Vaginal discharge

  - Skin infections

  - Gum infections

  - Mouth infections

  - Throat infection

  - Skin infections

  - Insect bites

18. Turkey Rhubarb – this herb is popularly known for its beneficial and positive effect on the digestive system. Even children can take advantage of the beneficial effects of this herb because it is gentle enough. In low doses, the roots can serve as an astringent tonic for better digestion while higher doses may be used as laxatives. In addition to this, turkey rhubarb is also known to treat the following:

  - Skin eruptions because of toxin accumulation

  - Menstrual problems

  - Hemorrhoids

  - Gall bladder problems

  - Liver diseases

  - Diarrhea

- Chronic constipation

19. Ginseng – is one of the most highly repudiated medicinal herbs in the orient. This wonder herb is touted for its ability to promote overall health, and general body vigor. The roots of this amazing medicinal plant is used to:

- Treat insomnia

- Address lack of appetite

- Treat debility related to old age

- Boost resistance against diseases

- Reduce levels of cholesterol

- Reduce blood sugar levels

- Enhance stamina

- Promote secretion of hormones

- Relax and stimulate the nervous system

20. Evening Primrose - the young roots of this medicinal plant can be consumed like a vegetable. The shoots may also be eaten as a salad. The roots of this wonder herb can be applied to bruises and piles. The roots may also be made into tea for the treatment of bowel pains and obesity. However, the more valuable parts are the bark and the leaves which are made into evening primrose oil, which is popularly known to treat the following conditions:

- Alcohol-associated liver damage

- Rheumatoid arthritis

- Brittle nails

- Acne

- Eczema

- Hyperactivity

- Premenstrual tension

- Multiple sclerosis

21. Tea tree – even the aborigines have utilized the leaves of tea tree for medicinal purposes, such as chewing fresh leaves to ease headaches. The

twigs, and leaves are made into tea tree oil which has antiseptic, antibacterial and antifungal properties. Tea tree oil definitely deserves a place in every household medicine cabinet. Tea tree oil is widely used for the treatment of the following illnesses:

- Minor burns

- Nits

- Cold sores

- Insect bites

- Warts

- Athlete's foot

- Acne

- Vaginal infections

- Thrush

- Chronic fatigue syndrome

- Glandular fever

- Cystitis

22. Great yellow gentian – the root of this powerful herb which is used to treat digestive problems. It is also capable of stimulating the digestive system, gallbladder and the liver. When taken internally, it is used to treat the following conditions:

- Anorexia

- Gastric infections

- Indigestion

- Liver complaints

Chapter 4: Know the Ten (10) Most Common Herb and Medicinal Garden Mistakes and How to Avoid Them

Common Mistake No. 1: Not applying any fertilizers.

Once you have herbs and medicinal plants planted and growing, it is very essential to keep them growing healthy with the use of a light, all purpose fertilizer. Apply a compost tea once every week to give your herbal and medicinal plants a boost. Herbs and medicinal plants are going to be harvested a lot of times during the growing season. This only means that your plants will be need an extra boost in order to keep their growth cycle for an extended time. When applying fertilizer, make sure to keep the soil hydrated and not the leaves themselves along with the compost tea. This practice will be healthier for the plant and contaminations in the leaves will also be avoided.

Common Mistake No. 2: Not protecting the plants enough.

While the herbal and medicinal plants are known to be hardy and resistant to diseases and bug problems, they can still arise. A lot of times, herbal and medicinal plant gardeners are scared to employ any strategy to safeguard their plants. This should not be the case. There are a lot of homemade and organic controls that are safe to use for edible herbal and medicinal plants. Organic gardening begins before the plant is even in place. Good soil and beneficial insects work altogether towards a chemical free herbal and medicinal garden.

Common Mistake No. 3: Not watering the plants properly

The needs of herbal and medicinal plants are very minimal. While they are very easy to maintain and care for, these plants will be providing you with fresh harvest all season. Herbal and medicinal plants however require proper watering schedule in order to remain free from stress.

Herbal and medicinal plants should be watered in the early morning, if possible. In this way, the water will soak deeper into the soil without having to deal with any evaporation issue. Always keep the soil around the plant hydrated and never water over the leaves as this will only promote diseases and mildews. Good mulch is important for your herbs as well. This will keep the soil hydrated and may extend the time between watering. Avoid mulching right next to the plant's stem though as this may invite insects and other types of invaders to make their home.

Common Mistake No. 4: Not paying attention to the tiny details.

It is a must to watch herbal and medicinal gardens closely. You need to know what the plant should look like while it is healthy as this will allow you to immediately notice when a problem first happens. Keep an eye on any damaged stems, leaves and disturbed soil around the plant. If you notice that the stems and leaves are beginning to fade, turn brown or curl up, you will have became aware of the problem early enough to possibly save the plant.

Common Mistake No. 4: Spraying chemical compounds into the plants

Herbs and medicinal plants are usually rinsed and used fresh. They should never be exposed to any kind of treatment that may possibly be toxic or dangerous to those who would eat them.

Even if a product claims that it is safe to use around pets and people, you should look for the words safe for edibles. You cannot rinse a bunch of basil leaves with water and soup prior to using. There are a lot of ways to keep ahead of the problems that may require the application of chemicals. Weed on a regular basis, watch the plants closely for any insect infestation and use natural fertilizers such as compost tea.

Common Mistake No. 5: Allowing the flowers to turn into seeds.

Herbal and medicinal plants grow beautiful flowers. While a lot of these plants have edible flowers, it is not a great idea to allow the herb to flower early during the growing season. Once your plant flowers, this signals that its life cycle is about to come into an end. Your plant is growing a flower, then a seed, then it dies back for that particular season.

It is a better idea to keep any blossoms from forming in the first place. When you see a flower about to grow, just pinch the entire thing off. You will notice that the plant may become persistent. In such case, cut the entire stem or below the flower.

Common Mistake No. 6: overcrowding or planting incorrectly

It is common to purchase more plants that you can possibly grow in a given area. When purchasing your herbal and medicinal plants, read the plant tags that usually come with each pot. Keep an eye to the width and height of the fully grown plant. You can always grow a quick growing annual between the plants, if you do not prefer the look of mulch. It is always a good idea to underplant rather than plant the herbs too close to each other from the beginning. Over planting is a big waste for money as it will not allow your plants to grow a healthy root system. A sturdy root system will help them survive the winter and expand the next growing season.

Common Mistake No. 7: Not cutting back enough

Pruning is what makes a plant to grow fast and neat. Pruning an herb implies that you are actually harvesting the good tasting stems and leaves. If you omit pruning, the plant will only tend to grow taller on a few stems. The leaves will grow old, dry and fall off. This will result to longer stems without leaves, Pruning will also allow the plant to begin and finish its life cycle. By regular pruning, you are actually keeping the plant in its growing phase for as long as possible. It will keep the flowers from budding, promotes leaves and stems and keeps the plant producing for an extended period of time. Your plants will appear healthier and better, if pruned back on a regular basis.

Common Mistake No. 9: Growing the plants in the wrong environment.

Are you growing rosemary, a chalky and dry loving plant in a humid and moist area? Your plant will surely die off in about 2 weeks from wet feet. If you would like to grow plants in a shady area, go for plants that can tolerate less sun. The sun=loving plants will grow weak and pale from not enough bright sunlight daily. If you have neither too shady nor too sunny area, try planting in pots that can be rolled or moved to the optimal lighting conditions. It is not a matter of sufficient shading or sun but is just a matter of finding a way to be adaptable to what you already have.

Common Mistake No. 10: Choosing unhealthy medicinal and herbal plants

The very first chance you have to find the perfect plant is when you actually buy it. Search for healthy plants, bright in color, plenty of foliage and certainly not one egg or bug on it. Finding a single aphid means that there are a lot more that you cannot see, all awaiting for the perfect time to invade your other plants. Never have the sympathy for a weak looking plant, unless you have a lot of space to keep it isolated from your main garden area while you try to repair the damage. The effort and time to be spent in repairing an infested herb garden means wasted time. Take the extra step to look for the healthiest plants that you can purchase.

Conclusion

Thank you again for purchasing this book!

I hope this book was able to help you to know how to successfully grow medicinal plants and herbs at home.

The next step is to follow the step-by-step guide and see your plants grow healthier each day.

Finally, if you enjoyed this book, please take the time to share your thoughts and post a review on Amazon. We do our best to reach out to readers and provide the best value we can. Your positive review will help us achieve that. It'd be greatly appreciated!

Thank you and good luck!

Check Out My Other Books

Below you'll find some of my other popular books that are popular on Amazon and Kindle as well. Simply click on the links below to check them out. Alternatively, you can visit my author page on Amazon to see other work done by me.

Coconut Oil for Easy Weight Loss

http://amzn.to/1i5f45p

Essential Oils & Aromatherapy

http://amzn.to/1ouuZTx

Superfoods that Kickstart Your Weight Loss

http://amzn.to/1eyHdku

The Best Secrets Of Natural Remedies

http://amzn.to/1gmHd7y

The Hypothyroidism Handbook

http://amzn.to/1emWfyR

The Hyperthyroidism Handbook

http://amzn.to/1kqLQCp

Essential Oils & Weight Loss For Beginners

http://amzn.to/Q83bFp

Essential Oils Box Set #30: Coconut Oil for Easy Weight Loss & The Beginners Guide to Medical Plants

Top Essential Oil Recipes

http://amzn.to/1lSrhSC

Soap Making For Beginners

http://amzn.to/1fkmYwr

Body Butters For Beginners

http://amzn.to/1fWjwJe

Homemade Body Scrubs & Masks For Beginners

http://amzn.to/1jjLRIO

Carrier Oils For Beginners

http://amzn.to/1sbqUQP

Natural Homemade Cleaning Recipes For Beginners

http://amzn.to/1izDB2m

The Beginners Guide To Medicinal Plants

http://amzn.to/1vSujr6

The Beginners Guide To Making Your Own Essential Oils

http://amzn.to/1piUNSB

The Beginners Alkaline Miracle Diet

http://amzn.to/1sDVaVE

**Essential Oils Box Set #30: Coconut Oil for Easy Weight Loss & The Beginners
Guide to Medical Plants**

Thyroid Diet

http://amzn.to/1piW2RY

Essential Oils Box Set #1 (Weight Loss + Essential Oil Recipes

http://amzn.to/1qlYWWP

Essential Oils Box Set #2 (Weight Loss + Essential Oil & Aromatherapy

http://amzn.to/1qlYWWP

Essential Oils Box Set #3 Coconut Oil + Apple Cider Vinegar

http://amzn.to/1oIFZJw

Essential Oils Box Set #4 Body Butters & Top Essential Oil Recipes

http://amzn.to/1jSxURJ

Essential Oils Box Set #5 Soap Making & Homemade Body Scrubs

http://amzn.to/RAvJYo

Essential Oils Box Set #6 Body Butters & Body Scrubs

http://amzn.to/RAvSel

Essential Oils Box Set #7 Top Essential Oils & Best Kept Secrets Of Natural
Remedies

http://amzn.to/1gvsRCq

Essential Oils Box Set #8 Homemade Cleaning Recipes & Essential Oil Recipes

http://amzn.to/1gxFAVb

Essential Oils Box Set #30: Coconut Oil for Easy Weight Loss & The Beginners Guide to Medical Plants

Essential Oils Box Set #9 Essential Oil and Weight Loss & Carrier Oils

http://amzn.to/1jmcEPP

Essential Oils Box Set #10 Hyperthyroidism Manual & Hypothyroidism Manual

http://amzn.to/1nHgJU4

Essential Oils Box Set #11 Carrier Oils for Beginners & Coconut Oil for Easy Weight Loss

http://amzn.to/1nHfy6X

Essential Oils Box Set #12 Essential Oils Weight Loss & Essential Oils Aromatherapy & Natural Homemade Cleaning Supplies & Top Essential Oil Recipes & Carrier Oils
http://amzn.to/1nHfy6X

Essential Oils Box Set #13 Superfoods & Essential Weight Loss & Essential Aromatherapy & Body Butters & Soap Making
http://amzn.to/1nUds6v

Essential Oils Box Set #14 Weight Loss & Apple Cider Vinegar & Body Butters & Homemade Body Scrubs & Coconut Oil for Beginners
http://amzn.to/1i1qYOd

If the links do not work, for whatever reason, you can simply search for these titles on the Amazon website to find them.

www.ingramcontent.com/pod-product-compliance
Lightning Source LLC
Chambersburg PA
CBHW070610290526
45790CB00002B/864